RECLAIMING YOUR LIFE AFTER A HYSTERECTOMY HEALING, INTIMACY, AND WELLNESS FOR WOMEN

Table of Contents

CHAPTER 1:

INTRODUCTION

Hi, I'm Aletta. I've been married for seven years, and I'm a proud mother of two beautiful children. The joy of my life is my two-year-old grandbaby, who lights up my world. While my family is the center of my heart, my health journey has shaped much of who I am today.

It has been a long and winding road, starting when I was just 17 years old. At that age, I had my first encounter with reproductive health issues—ovarian cysts that ruptured and led to a D&C (dilation and curettage) procedure. During that time, I found out I was pregnant with my first child, my beautiful daughter. Six years later, I welcomed my son into the world, and life seemed to move on smoothly. But my reproductive health story was far from over.

At the age of 22, during what I thought would be a routine check-up, I was diagnosed with multiple fibroids. The doctors reassured me there was nothing to worry about since the fibroids were the size of peas, and I, too, didn't think much of it at the time. However, as the years went by, my condition would take unexpected turns, and fibroids would become a defining part of my life.

In this book, I want to take you on a deeply personal journey, sharing my experiences of living with fibroids, how they impacted my daily life, and ultimately, my decision to undergo a robotic abdominal hysterectomy. It wasn't an easy choice, but it was necessary for my well-being, both physically and emotionally. The path to healing was not only about recovering from surgery but also about embracing a new chapter of life, learning to cope, and finding peace in my body's changes.

CHAPTER 2:

WHEN THE FIBROIDS TOOK OVER

By 2010, my fibroids had been part of my life for years, but they were still relatively manageable. They had grown, but not to the point where they seriously interfered with my daily activities. My doctor gave me clear advice on how to manage them: avoid caffeine, chocolate, and sugar, as these could stimulate further growth. For a long time, I stuck to that plan and managed to keep things under control. Life carried on, and I convinced myself that the fibroids would always just be a minor inconvenience.

But in 2013, things took a drastic turn. Out of nowhere, my periods became unbearably heavy, and I began to dread that time of the month. No matter how many pads I wore, I was constantly worried about leaking through my clothes. Doubling up, even tripling up, became my routine, but it didn't always work. There were days I would plan my entire schedule around my period, making sure I was near a restroom or somewhere private in case of an emergency. The fibroids were growing at a rapid pace, and I felt completely out of control of my own body. The emotional toll of constantly worrying about accidents and stains was overwhelming. I could no longer pretend that this was just a small issue I needed to take action.

Desperate to regain some control over my body, my husband and I decided to make a major lifestyle change. We went completely vegan, cutting out all meat, dairy, and processed foods. Our goal was not just weight loss, but healing. We even did a detox, which helped us shed 12 pounds in just two weeks. For the first time in a long time, I felt hopeful. My periods improved almost immediately they became lighter, less painful, and far more manageable. The results were so encouraging that I started to believe I had finally found the answer. I thought I had won the battle.

For six months, I stuck to the vegan lifestyle, and it truly felt like a turning point. I had more energy, I slept better, and most importantly, my fibroid symptoms were vastly reduced. My periods, which once left me bed-bound, became lighter and shorter. But like many lifestyle changes, maintaining that level of discipline was harder than I expected. The detox had been extreme, and over time, I found myself craving my old comforts, especially sugar.

It started small. A cookie here, a piece of chocolate there. But those indulgences began to snowball, and before I knew it, I had relapsed into my old habits. Chocolate chip cookies became my weakness, and even though I was still avoiding meat and dairy, the sugar cravings were powerful enough to bring back all of my old symptoms. My periods returned with a vengeance, becoming just as heavy and painful as before, if not worse. I remember feeling so defeated, as if all of my progress had been undone by just a few dietary slip-ups.

What made it worse was the realization that even though I had cut out meat and dairy, I hadn't entirely given up other indulgences, like shrimp. I convinced myself that seafood wouldn't have the same negative effects, but the truth was, my body needed a more drastic change.

The fibroids weren't going anywhere. No matter how much I tried to tweak my diet or detox, they remained a persistent presence in my life, reminding me that this was a much more complex battle than I had anticipated.

CHAPTER 3:

FIBROIDS AND INTIMACY

For years, fibroids were a manageable part of my life, and thankfully, they didn't interfere with my intimacy. My husband and I maintained a healthy, fulfilling sex life despite the occasional discomfort. But in 2018, everything changed. The fibroids, which had been quietly growing for years, suddenly took a turn for the worse.

The bleeding became unpredictable, often catching me off guard and leaving me anxious about when the next episode would strike. Sex, which had once been a source of connection and pleasure, became something I feared.

By 2020, my body had changed so much that I looked like I was nine months pregnant. The fibroids had grown rapidly, making me physically uncomfortable and emotionally drained. Intimacy with my husband became almost non-existent. It wasn't just the physical discomfort—there was also an overwhelming sense of embarrassment. I didn't feel like myself anymore. Every attempt at intimacy was overshadowed by the fear of bleeding or pain, and I couldn't shake the feeling of being trapped in a body that was betraying me. What once came naturally became an uphill battle.

This wasn't just a physical struggle; it was emotionally exhausting. My self-esteem plummeted, and I found myself sinking into a deep depression. Stress and anxiety became daily companions. I felt disconnected from myself, my body, and my husband. My libido had all but disappeared, and even though my husband was supportive and patient, I could see the toll it was taking on our relationship.

The fibroids had created a barrier between us—one that neither of us knew how to fully overcome.

At the same time, life wasn't slowing down to accommodate my physical or emotional challenges. By then, we had moved to South Carolina, and I was homeschooling our son while also running our trucking business from home. I was juggling so many responsibilities that it felt impossible to find time to take care of myself, let alone focus on my relationship. My body was telling me to slow down, but life doesn't always offer that option.

The combination of fibroids, depression, and the constant stress of everyday life had a profound impact on my quality of life. Intimacy became one of the many casualties. I felt isolated in my pain, as though I was watching my life unravel from the outside. Every day, I faced the reality that my health was slipping away, and with it, so many aspects of the life I once knew.

Fibroids weren't just affecting my body, they were affecting my marriage, my confidence, and my ability to find joy in the things that used to bring me happiness.

My health issues had turned my world upside down, and as much as I wanted to be the wife, mother, and business owner I had always been, the fibroids made me feel like a shell of my former self. I was constantly battling not only the physical symptoms but the emotional weight of feeling like I had lost control of my own life.

CHAPTER 4:

REACHING THE

BREAKING POINT

It wasn't until 2024 that I finally reached my breaking point. After years of living with fibroids and managing the constant discomfort, pain, and emotional toll, I realized I couldn't keep pretending that things would get better on their own. My periods, once merely heavy and inconvenient, had become a waking nightmare. They were now so excruciatingly painful and heavy that I could barely function during that time of the month. The unpredictability was crippling. I could no longer plan my life around the fibroids, they were controlling me.

My sex life, which had been steadily declining, was now almost non-existent. Every attempt at intimacy came with unbearable pain, which left me feeling broken, frustrated, and disconnected from my own body. The once small fibroids had grown into enormous, invasive masses, and I could no longer hide the effects they were having on my physical and emotional well-being. The stress and pain weighed on me like a constant shadow, and I knew something had to change. I couldn't live like this anymore.

I sought help from doctors once again. I had been through so many treatments—birth control pills, iron supplements to combat the relentless anemia from blood loss, and even painful injections meant to shrink the fibroids—but nothing worked. The fibroids only seemed to grow stronger, bigger, and more aggressive. I was losing hope with every failed treatment. Each doctor's visit seemed to end the same way: a temporary solution that never actually solved the problem.

By the time I went in for my third visit that year, I knew something drastic had to happen. During an ultrasound, the doctor revealed that I now had over

15 fibroids growing in my uterus. I was shocked. I knew they were big, but I hadn't realized just how out of control things had gotten. The largest fibroid weighed an astonishing 8 pounds; it was the size of a newborn baby! I felt like my body was no longer my own, as if these fibroids had taken over every part of my existence. The weight of them, both physically and emotionally, was too much to bear.

That moment was a turning point. I had no choice but to opt for a robotic abdominal hysterectomy. The thought of losing my uterus was difficult to process at first it's such a significant part of womanhood, of motherhood but I knew it was the only solution left. My health and quality of life were on the line, and I was done living in constant pain and fear. On May 6, 2024, I underwent the surgery that would change my life forever.

The hysterectomy was a complete success. My uterus, along with all the fibroids that had plagued me for so many years, were removed. As I woke up from surgery, I felt an overwhelming sense of relief wash over me. It wasn't just physical, it was emotional. For the first time in years, I felt like I could breathe again, like a weight had been lifted from my soul. The pain, the endless bleeding, the anxiety over my body betraying me all of it was gone.

It was one of the best decisions I ever made. Looking back, I can't believe I waited so long to take control of my health in this way. The surgery didn't just save me physically it gave me my life back. I could finally be present for my family, for my husband, and most importantly, for myself. The journey to that point had been long and painful, but in the end, it taught me how strong I truly was.

CHAPTER 5:

THE ROAD TO HEALING

Recovering from the hysterectomy was no walk in the park. The first few days were tough getting out of bed felt like a monumental task, and my body was sore in ways I hadn't expected. But I knew I had made the right decision, and I was determined to heal. Every day, despite the pain, I made a conscious effort to get out of bed and keep moving. Even when it hurt, I reminded myself that this was part of the process. Healing takes time, but I wasn't going to let it defeat me.

Nutrition became a major focus in my recovery. I had always known that what we eat plays a huge role in how our bodies function, but during this time, it became clearer than ever. My meals became simple but nutrient-packed. I relied heavily on fruit smoothies. They were easy to prepare, refreshing, and filled with vitamins to help my body rebuild. They became my go-to, especially on days when my appetite wasn't the greatest.

I also made a conscious effort to cut out caffeine, knowing it could slow down my healing. Instead, I focused on incorporating greens and protein-rich foods like quinoa and broccoli. This vegetarian approach wasn't just about healing my body—it was about regaining my energy. I wanted to fuel myself with foods that would support my recovery and get me back to feeling like myself again. I knew that eating clean and nourishing my body from the inside out was the key to getting stronger each day.

It wasn't easy, but I started to notice small improvements with every passing week. My energy slowly began to return, and I found myself able to move around more freely. The pain, which had once felt all-consuming, was gradually fading into the background. I could finally focus on life again, not just on the physical toll that the fibroids had taken on me. It felt like I was getting my freedom back, one step at a time.

Six weeks after the surgery, I went in for my post-op appointment, anxious but hopeful. I had followed the doctor's instructions diligently, prioritizing rest and giving my body the space it needed to heal. When my doctor told me I had healed impeccably, it was the validation I needed. I walked out of that office feeling lighter, as though a huge burden had been lifted from my shoulders. The pain that had haunted me for so many years was finally gone.

I felt like a new woman pain-free, energized, and ready to reclaim my life. For the first time in years, I could see a future that wasn't overshadowed by fibroids, bleeding, or exhaustion. My body had gone through a lot, but it had also proven its resilience. This journey wasn't just about removing fibroids; it was about rediscovering my strength, my health, and my sense of self.

CHAPTER 6:
RECLAIMING INTIMACY AFTER SURGERY

Let's talk about sex after a hysterectomy. For many women, the idea of resuming intimacy after surgery can be daunting. The fear of pain, the changes in your body, and the emotional toll of everything you've been through can make it feel intimidating. I've been there, and I understand how it feels. But here's the good news: you can absolutely get your sex life back on track, and in my experience, it can be even better than before.

The key to reclaiming intimacy after surgery is patience and positioning. Your body needs time to heal, and it's important to listen to it. The first few times may feel different, and that's okay. Take it slow, and don't rush yourself. Your comfort is the most important thing. Over time, you'll rediscover the pleasure and connection that comes with intimacy, and you might be surprised at how much your body can still enjoy these moments.

One of the most helpful things I discovered was finding positions that reduce discomfort and allowed me to experience pleasure more fully. For me, elevating my legs was a game-changer. When your legs are raised to your partner's shoulder height, it takes some of the pressure off your pelvic area, making things feel much more comfortable. Another position that worked for me was holding one leg up while keeping the other flat this gave me more control over the pressure and intensity.

These small adjustments made all the difference. I could ease into things without worrying about pain, and over time, I felt more confident. It wasn't just about reducing discomfort; it was about opening myself up to feeling pleasure in a new way. The intimacy I shared with my husband became deeper, more meaningful, and surprisingly, more enjoyable than it had been in years.

CHAPTER 7:

DIET AND HEALING

A plant-based, vegetarian diet can work wonders for your recovery after surgery. Throughout my healing journey, I discovered just how powerful food can be when it comes to rebuilding your body from the inside out. After my hysterectomy, I made a conscious decision to focus on nutrient-rich, healing foods, and the difference it made was incredible.

During those crucial weeks of recovery, I filled my meals with leafy greens, quinoa, broccoli, and fresh fruit. These foods are packed with vitamins, minerals, and antioxidants that help your body repair and regain strength. Leafy greens like spinach and kale became staples in my diet, providing essential nutrients like iron and calcium. Quinoa and broccoli, on the other hand, became my go-to sources of protein and fiber, keeping me full and energized without feeling heavy or sluggish.

One of the most significant changes I made was cutting out sugar, dairy, and caffeine. Before the surgery, I often relied on coffee and sugary treats to get through the day, but I soon realized that these were only draining my energy and worsening my symptoms. By eliminating them from my diet, I noticed an immediate improvement in my energy levels, digestion, and overall well-being. It was as if my body was finally able to focus on healing instead of constantly fighting against the effects of unhealthy foods.

This shift to a plant-based, whole-food diet wasn't just about avoiding things that could slow my recovery—it was about fueling my body with everything it needed to heal faster and more effectively. Every bite I took felt like a step toward reclaiming my health, and it empowered me to take control of my recovery.

Smoothies became a staple during this time, especially on days when I didn't feel like eating much. I would blend up nutrient-packed fruit smoothies with spinach, berries, bananas, and chia seeds to ensure I was still getting the vitamins I needed to stay strong. These smoothies were easy to digest and gave me a quick boost of energy when I needed it most.

Choosing a plant-based diet during my recovery wasn't just about physical healing—it also had a profound impact on my mental and emotional well-being. As my body grew stronger and healthier, I felt more in tune with myself. I regained the energy I had been missing for so long and felt more vibrant than I had in years.

This journey taught me that what you put into your body matters, especially when you're healing. By focusing on nourishing, plant-based foods, you can help your body recover more efficiently, reduce inflammation, and regain your strength. The road to healing isn't just about rest and medical treatment—it's about fueling yourself with the right ingredients for a healthy, vibrant future.

CHAPTER 8:

FINAL THOUGHTS

I hope my story encourages you to take control of your health and your life. A hysterectomy doesn't have to be the end of anything, it can actually be the beginning of a fresh start. I know firsthand how overwhelming it can feel, from the pain, the uncertainty, to the fear of what life might look like afterward. But I want you to know that with patience, care, and a deep focus on your body's needs, you can heal, reclaim your strength, and experience life fully once again.

For me, this journey wasn't just about surgery, it was about transformation. I learned to listen to my body in ways I hadn't before. The surgery didn't just remove the fibroids that were weighing me down; it allowed me to rediscover my sense of well-being. It showed me that healing is possible, and that life after a hysterectomy can be vibrant, intimate, and fulfilling.

Every woman's body is unique, and so is every woman's journey. What worked for me may not look the same for you, but that's okay. The key is to trust your body and give it the time it needs to recover. Be kind to yourself throughout this process. Healing isn't always linear, and there will be ups and downs. But through it all, you are strong, capable, and worthy of feeling good again.

Don't rush your journey, but also don't shy away from taking control of your health. You deserve to feel strong and healthy, and you deserve to live without the constant pain and discomfort that fibroids or other conditions may bring. The path to reclaiming your life starts now, and it's a path you can walk with confidence.

You are more powerful than you know. This is your chance to put yourself first, to listen to your body, and to nurture it with the care and patience it needs.

Your health, your intimacy, and your joy don't have to be sacrificed. They can thrive, and you can too.

CHAPTER 9:

THANK YOU

Thank you for taking the time to read my story and this guide. If there's one thing I hope you take away from this book, it's this: your health matters. Don't wait until things are unbearable before you take action, stay on top of your checkups, listen to your body, and prioritize your well-being.

I made the mistake of waiting 14 years before truly addressing my fibroids, and in that time, my quality of life suffered. Ignoring the signs only prolonged my pain and discomfort. I want you to know that you don't have to go through the same struggle. Your health is worth fighting for, and you deserve to live a life that's free of pain and full of happiness.

So, whether you're facing fibroids or another health issue, take the time to care for yourself, make decisions that are right for you, and never ignore what your body is trying to tell you. You are worthy of feeling good and living your best life.

Until next time, keep shining bright!